THE DIY MEGA FOODS PLAN

EAT SIMPLY. LIVE FULLY.

BY ANDREW TAYLOR & MANDY VAN ZANEN

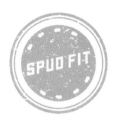

OUR OTHER BOOKS

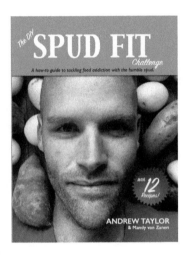

The DIY Spud Fit Challenge

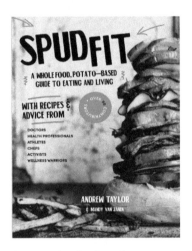

Spud Fit: A whole food, potato-based guide to eating and living.

Learn more about our courses, community and coaching at

www.spudfit.com

email: andrew@spudfit.com

Food photography and styling by Paula Banda: www.anewgreenleaf.com.
Edited by Amanda Holder: amandaholdereditingservices@gmail.com.
Cover design and typesetting by Nikka Ojela Guadalupe.

DISCLAIMER

I am not a doctor, nor do I claim to be any kind of health expert. The information contained in these pages is the result of my own research as a layperson, and of my direct personal experiences. If you choose to follow the information here, you should do so under the supervision of your doctor. This is especially important if you are on any medication - it is quite common for health to improve so rapidly and dramatically on a whole foods, plant-based regime that continuing to take some medications can become dangerous.

TABLE OF CONTENTS

INTRO

In February of 2016 my story went viral. After a month of eating nothing but potatoes and losing 10 kilograms (22 pounds) in the process, I became a global freak show. I was the butt of jokes and internet memes everywhere and "experts" were coming out of the woodwork to predict my demise.

A few months earlier I'd realised that food addiction was the root of all my weight gain and health problems. Logic dictated that I should treat my problem with the same gold standard treatment we apply to almost every other addiction - the abstinence model. We can all agree that cigarette, drugs and alcohol and gambling addicts do best if they quit entirely, whereas food addicts are constantly told to eat 'everything in moderation'. I had tried and failed at moderation on a daily basis for most of my life and I was ready to smash that idea to pieces.

I figured that if I focused first and foremost on getting my addiction under control, then I might, finally, be able to stick with a more well-rounded, sustainable healthy eating plan that actually worked. To cut a long story (and a lot of research) short, I ate nothing but potatoes for all of 2016. More importantly, in the process I totally changed my relationship with food and rebuilt myself as a 'new' person from the ground up. As an added bonus, I lost around 55kg (121lbs) for the year and was no longer suffering with clinical depression and anxiety. All of my blood tests improved throughout the year, my long- term problems with irritable bowel syndrome went away and my doctor could not have been happier with the state of my health. My passion to help others enjoy the same success was born.

Media outlets followed my progress throughout the year and, as I changed before their eyes, so did the opinions of their so-called "experts".

The Spud Fit Challenge started as a purely selfish experiment and has since grown into a movement, changing the lives of literally tens of thousands of people all around the world. The most important thing about the Spud Fit Challenge is what you do when it's over. In fact the whole reason I came up with the Spud Fit Challenge at all was to help me realign my thoughts, feelings and actions around food so I'd be able to stick with healthy eating habits in the long term once my year of spuds was over. I'd tried and failed at adopting a healthy whole foods plant-based (WFPB) diet many times. The Spud Fit Challenge was my way to "break glass in case of emergency" and hit the reset button on my relationship with food. I've since been able to stick with my version of a WFPB diet which I call the Mega Foods Plan. The Spud Fit Challenge is what made that possible for me.

It's now five years since I finished my year-long Spud Fit challenge and the two most common questions I get are:

1. Do you still eat only potatoes? (No)
2. Well then what do you eat?

If what comes next is the most important part, then this book is long overdue and even more crucial than our first book, The DIY Spud Fit Challenge.

The Mega Foods Plan is also a stand-alone program. Starting with mega foods, rather than just potatoes, is an excellent plan that you can stick with forever. Many people have had great success doing just that.

The question of "What do you eat?" in most cases is actually code for "What should I eat?" This is a very simple question and it has a very simple answer. The simplest answer I can give is—plants. I eat *a lot* of plants.

My aim for this book is to have that answer make sense to you by the time you finish reading.

WHY DO WE NEED
THE MEGA FOODS PLAN?

The meat industry wants us to believe we need more protein and iron. The dairy industry wants us to believe we need more calcium. The egg industry wants us to believe that cholesterol is not that bad after all. The seafood industry wants us to believe we need more omega 3s. The olive and coconut oil industries want us to believe we need more "good fats". The junk food industry wants us to believe we should eat "everything in moderation". The pharmaceutical industry wants us to believe that they have more power over our health than we do. Reality cooking shows want us to believe that every meal should be a gourmet extravaganza. Supplement and superfood companies want us to believe we are in imminent danger of being deficient in everything and that no matter how much of a given nutrient we consume, more will always be better. The only reason these beliefs are so ubiquitous is because a lot of corporate bank accounts depend on it.

Some scientists, doctors and health professionals do their best to make sure we know the truth about good nutrition. Others are heavily influenced by vested interests in the aforementioned industries, to share a message that flies in the face of broadly accepted scientific evidence. This serves to keep us confused and held hostage by indecision.

The Mega Foods Plan is my attempt to cut through the chaos, simplify food and bring the focus back to what's always been most important when it comes to our health and well-being: eating well.

There are many healthy whole food plant based eating plans that will bring great results if you can stick with them. The key word here is "if". A major focus of our Mega Foods Plan is on making healthy eating as simple and easy as possible to follow. I hope the following pages will set you up to make consistent good decisions and develop new habits around food that will stick with you through even the most stressful times.

THE PROBLEM WITH SUPERFOODS

Don't get me wrong here, spirulina and goji berries truly are great! It's all well and good to aim for the best of everything and there's nothing inherently wrong with superfoods. They just don't deserve so much attention.

As a society we focus relentlessly on getting more, more, more of anything that is deemed to be good. More protein, more calcium, more vitamins, more minerals, more antioxidants. Because if these things are healthy then more of them must be more healthy, right? No matter how good our diet is, there is always pressure for us to make it better. In our quest for endless improvement, we turn to superfoods with their marketing hype that promise bigger, better, stronger, higher, faster health.

Typical superfoods tend to be expensive, hard to find, taste like crap and do nothing to satisfy hunger. They don't provide the necessary energy to fuel a busy day, but they do allow us to feel like we are doing something positive for our health, without actually doing much at all. A family member once told me that he didn't need to worry about changing his diet to bring his cholesterol down because drugs were already doing that for him. Superfoods have assumed a similar role in the lives of many, providing us with an opportunity to have our cake and eat it too.

Superfoods give us a false sense of security. You wouldn't hang a beautiful painting on a cracked wall. You wouldn't put a turbocharger on a misfiring engine. You wouldn't plant roses in a garden overrun by weeds. We need to accept that a blend of exotic powders and a shaker bottle cannot offset the cookies we allow ourselves for a special treat because we really deserve it... six times a week. If your weekends are full of pizza and ice cream then you shouldn't concern yourself with superfoods on Monday morning.

THE PROBLEM WITH SUPERFOODS

Get the basics right first. Fix the wall, tune the engine, weed the garden and ditch the junk foods. When your car is purring like a kitten and chewing up the open road without a second thought, then you can consider adding a turbo charger.

WHAT ARE MEGA FOODS?
WHY ARE THEY GOOD?

Mega Foods are the staples that have helped billions of our ancestors thrive throughout all of our documented history. In fact recent studies of bacteria found on ancient neanderthal teeth have shown that six hundred thousand years ago, the diet of our ancestors centred on starchy, carbohydrate-rich foods. Contrary to the popular belief that meat eating gave us big brains, learning to cook grains, legumes and tubers is what suddenly gave us access to an abundant supply of glucose that fuelled the growth of the human brain. It appears that hunter-gatherers placed a great emphasis on the gathering!

The ancient Egyptians, Greeks and Romans based their diet on grains and legumes. Rice was so important that it was actually used as currency in Japan and China, and it remains a staple throughout Asia. Potatoes played a large part in the success of the ancient South Americans of Inca and Machu Picchu. To this day, the healthiest, longest lived populations on earth get the majority of their calories from Mega Foods.

In many ways Mega Foods are the antithesis of superfoods. They're cheap, simple, easy, delicious, hearty and satisfying! They are easy to grow and you can always find them in any local grocery store or on the menu of any restaurant, cafe or takeaway store. A major key to the success of the Mega Foods Plan is that it can provide you with enough energy to power through your day, while simultaneously making it very difficult to overeat and gain fat (see the calorie density section of this book to learn why).

Okay, get to the point Andrew, what ARE Mega Foods?!

WHAT ARE MEGA FOODS?
WHY ARE THEY GOOD?

It's pretty simple really—Mega Foods are whole, unprocessed grains, legumes and starchy tubers. Think of grains like rice, oats, wheat, barley, millet, quinoa, bulgur and corn. Legumes like peas, all types of beans, chickpeas and lentils. Tubers include many different types of potatoes and sweet potatoes.

I also like to think of the more calorie-dense fruits as honorary Mega Foods. While they don't necessarily have the same level of importance in human history as our starchy foods, they can play a very important role in our lives right now. I love fruits like bananas, apples, mangoes, melons, grapes and citrus fruits for their similar ability to hit that slightly higher calorie density sweet spot where we can get enough energy to thrive, but not enough to gain fat. These 'mega fruits' are nature's fast food, which is the main reason I think they're so important. They're perfect for on-the-go snacks (or even entire meals) when you aren't prepared or don't have time to cook mega foods.

An equally important question is - what AREN'T mega foods? Which foods should we avoid when following the Mega Foods Plan?

This is also pretty simple: processed foods and animal foods are not part of the Mega Foods Plan. These foods are devoid of fibre and are far lower in many vitamins, minerals and antioxidants. Their lack of fibre and water content makes them very high in calorie density too, which makes them hard to stop eating and contributes to rapid weight gain and inflammation among other things.

Meat is an extremely valuable food for hunter-gatherer populations of past and present, whose primary concern is obtaining enough calories to survive. With an abundance of calories available to us at any time, we need to flip our thinking in line with the calorie density model.

WHAT ARE MEGA FOODS?
WHY ARE THEY GOOD?

We'll get to all this in more detail later.

No oil!

Oil gets a special mention here because it's so commonly thought of as a health food. I want to take a moment to dispel that myth right now. Oil is a highly processed food, with no fibre and negligible nutritional value. It's 100% pure fat, which is the most highly concentrated calorie source available to us.

If you take some sugar cane and remove the fibre, protein and water along with most of the vitamins and minerals, then you're left with sugar. We all agree that this is a processed food that's very unhealthy and best left out of our diet or at least kept to a minimum.

On the other hand you can go through a very similar level of processing with an olive - remove the fibre, carbohydrate and water along with most of the vitamins and minerals, then you're left with olive oil. Somehow we're led to believe that this results in a health food that we should buy in gallon bottles to pour over our salads and add to just about everything we cook.

I can hear the chorus of voices right now yelling "What about the Mediterranean diet?!" It's true that there are many studies showing that when people switch to a Mediterranean style diet, which includes olive oil, they tend to get healthier and lose weight. However, this happens in spite of the oil, not because of it. The Mediterranean diet includes plenty of fresh vegetables, fruit, grains and beans while excluding processed foods (other than oil) and limiting animal foods. This is certainly an improvement on the standard western diet, which is reflected in the results of diet studies. You'll see plenty of headlines spruiking olive oil as being a healthy option, but in reality they only show that olive oil is better than other oils. I'm yet to see even a single study showing that any kind of oil might be better than no oil at all.

Rules create friction, pressure and stress. Most diet plans out there have a bunch of rules that we need to follow to be successful. There are rules about what kinds of foods to eat, how much, what time of day, how often, how many times we should chew, etc. More rules around what type of hunger you should listen to, what kinds of foods you should keep in the house, how you should do your shopping and prepare your meals. Rules for how big your plate should be and what percentages of your plate should contain certain foods. The list of dieting rules I've tried to follow could go on and on!

More rules = more opportunities to fail

The daily grind eventually wears us down until we can't handle it anymore and, shock horror, we end up swallowing our food after twenty-six chews instead of forty-five! This in itself is no big deal, except that this perceived failure kills our self esteem, which triggers a negative spiral. Before we know it, the floodgates open, we're breaking all the rules and the weight starts to pile back on.

While we do need to have some rules, I think it's very important to get rid of as many as possible. Fewer rules mean less friction, less pressure and less stress. It also guarantees fewer chances to fail. I've boiled the Mega Foods Plan down to a few key rules:

THE RULES

1) Eat as much as you feel like, as often as you feel like it.

I've left the word hunger out of this rule on purpose because it's irrelevant. Please don't go turning this rule into "eat only when you're hungry" or some seasoned-dieter variation on that. It's ok to eat because you're stressed, tired, bored, anxious, depressed or all of the above. It's also ok to eat in between meals, after 8pm or even after bed. If you want a snack at 3 am, go for it! It's ok to have second helpings. It's even ok to have an entire extra meal! Don't overthink it, just eat when you feel like eating and stop when you feel like stopping. Over time, your brain and gut will work together to adjust your hunger drive according to your actual physiological needs. Your body knows exactly what to do. It just needs you to get out of the way!

Skip ahead to the section on calorie density for the nuts and bolts on why you really can eat as much as you want, whenever you want!

2) Eat plants, emphasise starch

If it's an unprocessed plant food - eat it. If it isn't - don't. Put your emphasis on starchy mega foods. It really is that simple!

You don't need to eat specific amounts of anything and you don't need to track, measure, weigh, log or count anything at all.

Eat as many colourful veggies, fruits and mushrooms as you want. Add flavour with onion, garlic and as many fresh or dried herbs and spices as you want.

Keep your focus on potatoes, sweet potatoes, whole grains and legumes to make sure you're getting good, clean, efficient energy to power your day and keep you feeling full and satisfied. Personally, I like to focus mostly on potatoes and sweet potatoes, but if you prefer rice and beans or a combination of all starches, that's fine too!

THE RULES

3) Medical supervision

It goes without saying, but I'll say it anyway: all major diet and lifestyle changes should be done with the supervision of your doctor. Many medications (especially those for blood pressure and diabetes) can become dangerous if you continue to take them when they're no longer needed.

Besides that, data can give you positive feedback on your progress. It's nice to see the number on the scales go down but it's even better to see your blood pressure and cholesterol normalise and your medications reduce.

4) No more rules!

Seriously, you don't need any more rules than the ones outlined above. It's very tempting to add your own little tweaks and modifications to any plan. You can speed things up for yourself by adjusting certain aspects, but at the same time you can add more pressure, more stress and more opportunities to fail and throw in the towel.

Keep it simple, keep your focus narrow. Follow these four rules and everything will work out just fine.

SIMPLE MEAL PLANNING

Eat and repeat

The point of this concept is to reduce the amount of thinking and planning that goes into your food. Make your decisions ahead of time and get in a comfortable routine that allows you to enjoy your food without being obsessed with it. Choose a handful of meals that are quick and easy to make, that you enjoy eating and that fit in with your lifestyle. Write yourself a menu and eat those meals on high rotation! Pick one or two meals that you are happy with for breakfast, another one or two for lunch and the same again for dinner. EXPERT TIP: You can eat 'dinner foods' for breakfast and 'breakfast foods' for dinner - good foods are edible at all times of the day!

Decide on your meals for the coming week (or longer) and get comfortable with eating the same meals over and over again. As you progress you can sub different meals in and out of the rotation.

When you cook, make a huge batch so you can store leftovers and have quick meals for the next couple of days.

WHAT TO EXPECT

If you've started with your own Spud Fit Challenge, then the first and most obvious consideration is figuring out when to make the switch to the Mega Foods Plan. The Spud Fit Challenge can be hard in the beginning for many of us. Thoughts, cravings and even dreams of other foods can be overwhelming at times. As we keep walking the path, putting one foot in front of the other, we find that it gets much easier. Most people eventually come to a place where they're no longer bothered by cravings and desires to eat other foods. In fact most people get to the point where they're pretty comfortable eating only potatoes and aren't really bothered by thoughts of what they'd rather be eating.

I think when you reach that point where you're no longer fantasising about what that first non-potato meal might be, that's a good time to start planning your transition to Mega Foods. When other foods don't have that same pull anymore, then the challenge to maintain control will be less intense.

Start slowly, add one new food at a time. Begin with other foods that you find boring. Broccoli is a favourite for this process because it's relatively uninspiring and is unlikely to result in you locking yourself in the pantry, hiding from your family, while you inhale your secret stash of steamed florets.

After a couple of days of spuds and broccoli, try adding tomatoes for a little more flavour. A couple of days after that you might add in a fruit like bananas. Take this process seriously and do it slowly so that you can develop a true awareness of how these foods affect you both physically and mentally. Use your own judgement and keep adding simple, unprocessed plant foods as you feel comfortable. Maintain your focus on simple, repetitive eating while getting the most out of life.

WHAT TO EXPECT

If you're coming to the Mega Foods Plan as your first foray into the world of plant based eating rather than as a follow on from a Spud Fit Challenge, you'll likely encounter some 'detox' symptoms along the way. I don't like the word 'detox' for this process because the body is excellent at detoxing and is always doing it 24/7. I think a better term for this is "adjustment". You can't send a memo to your digestive system ahead of time, warning it of what's coming and encouraging it to be prepared. You just have to start your new diet and then wait for your body to play catch-up. You won't be used to eating this way and, therefore, your digestive system won't be set up to deal with it efficiently and extract all you need from this new fuel. It'll take a while to clean out your system and grow a new gut microbiome that thrives on premium fuel. Be patient.

WHERE DO YOU GET YOUR...?

When I ate a steady diet of pizza, ice cream and chocolate, I never gave a second thought to making sure I got enough of x, y or z nutrients. That concern only came when I stopped eating all that crap!

If there's one thing that most humans do need more, more, more of, it's fibre! Study after study consistently shows strong correlations between fibre intake and positive health outcomes. Populations who eat more fibre have lower rates of heart disease, cholesterol, hypertension, diabetes, stroke, osteoporosis, breast cancer, bowel cancer and several other cancers too. This list could go on and on, suffice to say that people who eat more fibre from whole, unprocessed foods tend to not only have more years in their life but also more life in their years.

Gut health has become a major focus in recent years, which has fuelled the sales of probiotic pills, powders and potions. The problem with this approach is that it's largely pointless to add billions of healthy bugs to your digestive system if they're just going to starve to death when they get there. Mega Foods provide plenty of delicious prebiotic fibre to feed the healthy bacteria and keep your little friends happy and thriving. With the possible exception of recovering from a dose of antibiotics, you don't need to spend your hard-earned money on probiotic supplements, you just need to create an environment in which they will naturally thrive. It's important to note that fibre supplements don't have the same positive impact. Metamucil or psyllium husk can help in certain situations but they're no substitute for the fabulous fibre in a bowl of beans, rice and veggies. If you build it, they will come!

WHERE DO YOU GET YOUR...?

Where do you get your protein?

Protein is made up of amino acids. When we eat meat, we get protein, which the body then has to break down into amino acids. These amino acids are reassembled into the specific types of proteins that we need, depending on the job that needs to be done.

The good news is that every single unprocessed plant food available to us contains all the required amino acids for our body to create every kind of protein we need. Despite the constant fear mongering, there is no 'protein deficiency' ward at your local hospital. If we are eating enough food then we are getting enough protein: it really is that simple! How do you know if you're eating enough food? If you're following our rules and eating as much as you feel like, as often as you feel like it, then you're good to go. Now I'd really like you to forget you ever heard the word protein!

Where do you get your calcium?

Chalk is mostly made of calcium and I certainly would not trust that with taking the impact of a strong tackle in a football game! Could you imagine a kid jumping down from the monkey bars and relying on bones made of chalk to break their fall? The dairy industry would love you to believe that high calcium intake is all you need for strong bones, but there's much more to it than that.

Despite the decades-long scare campaign, it's actually quite easy to get more than enough calcium. There's plenty of calcium in beans and legumes, dark leafy greens and other veggies, cruciferous veggies and nuts and seeds. Some grains and fruits are also good sources. In fact I'd argue that if you follow the Mega Foods Plan, it's almost impossible not to get enough calcium.

WHERE DO YOU GET YOUR...?

Just like with building muscle, strong bones develop as a result of the stress you put them under. Your muscles grow stronger because you work them hard and your bones are no different.

Where do you get your iron?

Shortly after my year of eating only potatoes ended, I was invited by the South Australian Potato Board to speak at a farming exhibition. I didn't realise that a lot of people in the room were cow farmers until question time, when a proud cow farmer stood up and said, "surely without eating any meat, your iron levels would've gotten dangerously low by the end of the year?". I told him that when eating only potatoes, I was actually getting way more than my recommended daily intake of iron. I also told him that at my last medical check-up, my doctor said that the oxygen-carrying my blood's oxygen levels were almost as high as blood-doping athletes at the Tour de France! The cow farmers in the audience were less than happy with that answer. The truth is that it just couldn't be easier to get enough iron on the Mega Foods Plan. Eat plenty, or planty (haha!) of spuds, legumes, veggies and fruits, and you can't go wrong.

What you don't eat is far more important than what you do

I desperately want you to forget about getting enough or more of any individual nutrient. I want you to forget you ever heard of protein or calcium or vitamins or minerals or anything else. I want you to put your full energy and focus into simply making sure you don't eat any of the crap that causes problems. If you don't eat junk, then you don't need to eat anything specific to counteract the problems caused by junk. When you remove the calorie-dense, fibre-deficient and micronutrient-deficient foods from your diet, then all that's left is the right choice. First, do no harm.

HELPFUL HINTS

Making changes is hard. Getting out of your comfort zone is hard. A big reason most people regain any weight they lose is because eating well can also be very hard if you let it. The following hints and tips are aimed at helping you to make this as easy as possible, so that you can make the healthy choice the easy choice. A small change in the way you physically and mentally navigate certain situations can go a long way towards making long-term success easy.

Get support: People who run with a group are usually better runners than those who don't. People who play in a band or orchestra are usually better musicians than those who don't. Your chances of long-term success increase if you surround yourself with like-minded people who are working towards the same goal. This doesn't mean you should cut certain people out of your life, but you could make an effort to get to know some healthy people. Many cities have meet-up groups that gather to share healthy meals and experiences. There are many online groups that are very helpful with sharing ideas including, of course, our Spud Fit online group— the most supportive and lovely group on the internet! Join for free at www.spudfit.com

Eating out: The most important thing is to eat before you go. I'm not talking about a snack as you head out the door either; I mean have a full meal before you go out to eat. When you've already eaten, it's much easier to make healthy choices. More importantly, it's much easier to focus your attention on the people you love and be fully engaged with the conversation when you're not so easily distracted by food.

It's also a good idea to look at the menu online before you go, so you can have your decision already made when you get to the restaurant. You can even call ahead to check. That way you don't even have to look at the menu with all its temptations. In the past I've ordered steamed, boiled or baked potatoes or rice (no added oil), steamed veggies, large salads with balsamic vinegar, grilled veggies, pasta with veggies. Add salt and pepper to spice it up.

HELPFUL HINTS

Be a scientist: Imagine you're part of a scientific experiment where people are studying the effects of following the Mega Foods Plan for a month. A good impartial scientist would not be emotionally invested in getting a positive or negative outcome, they'd just want to find out what happens. This scientist wouldn't get excited at a weight loss on day two and they wouldn't get upset about a weight gain on day seven. They'd simply write the numbers down on their chart and carry on with the experiment because they know that they can't make any judgements until the month is over and they've had a chance to analyse the data. Try to see yourself as the scientist. You're not in it for the daily ups and downs, you're in it for the long haul so that you can really find out what happens if you stick with it. You'll never know the results if you don't run the experiment!

Cooking without oil: I know it sounds weird and you think it's not possible, but I promise you it is! You don't need oil to stop onion from sticking to a fry pan, you just need a splash of water. A good quality non-stick pan helps too but it's not necessary. Just make sure you get your pan hot before you add the food and then use a little water to keep it from sticking. It will feel strange at first and it will take some getting used to, but your waistline and blood pressure will thank you for it!

Frozen, canned, pre-packed foods: Cooking everything from scratch is a nice idea but I've rarely got time for that! Pre-cut frozen veggies have been a lifesaver for us and we now use them every day. A teaspoon of already crushed garlic from a jar with a handful of frozen chopped onion is so fast! Combine that with a bag of chopped frozen mixed veggies, a can of beans and a bag of pre-cooked rice and you've got a super healthy, delicious meal on the table in under ten minutes. Don't let all these crazy TV cooking shows fool you: cooking is not a competition. Just do what you have to do to get a decent meal on the table and in your belly.

HELPFUL HINTS

If fancy yourself as a master chef this might be something you'd rather not hear: now might be the time to consider whether your culinary ways are helping or hindering your real goals for wellbeing. Embrace our new way for now and see where it leads.

Prior preparation prevents poor performance: Meal prep is the last thing I want to do on a Sunday afternoon. I feel sick when I see Instagram pics of a hundred containers all lined up on the bench with various meals, snacks and other concoctions for the week. I have nothing in common with people who do this and I hope I never get stuck talking to them at a party! I like to keep my meal prep simple. I always have a box of cooked spuds and a box of cooked rice in the fridge, ready to heat and eat. Often there's a box of cooked beans in there too. It's easy to put on a pot of Mega Foods to cook while I'm doing other things. I set a timer on my watch so I don't get distracted and leave it for too long (I learned that one the hard way).

Free food mentality: Free lunch at work, doughnuts at church, barbecue after the sports game. It's really hard to say no to free food, especially when it's exciting, delicious and shared with friends. Well, nothing in life comes for free. Junk food will be paid for with your health and happiness. Fill up on Mega Foods to turn down the volume on your cravings and then turn your focus to enjoying the company of the people around you.

Cooking for others: Ideally, you could have a conversation with your supportive family and they could either start cooking their own meals or eat the healthy mega foods that you make. If this is not realistic for you, then you can plan your way through it. Eat before you start cooking other foods - it's much easier to resist when you aren't hungry. Have healthy food with you while you're cooking, so you can easily grab a mouthful here and there to keep you going. Ask others to do taste tests for you. With some pre-planning, cooking tempting foods is not a surprise that sneaks up on you. Plan for it and you can find a way to make the situation work.

What should I eat for breakfast? This is one of the most common questions I hear. All foods are edible at all times of the day and night. You don't need breakfast or lunch or snack ideas. These are just cultural habits; stories that you've been told and you're now telling yourself. You're allowed to have a stir-fry for breakfast and porridge for dinner. You're also allowed to have a bowl of soup as a snack. No matter what time it is, just eat some food that you enjoy and move on with your day!

Make your food boring and your life interesting: This is something I've said a lot. That doesn't mean you shouldn't enjoy your food or do anything that might make it taste nicer, it's just an acknowledgement that it's ok to eat food that's not as exciting as we are used to. It's about being aware that getting too much excitement, emotional support, comfort and enjoyment from food is what got us into this mess in the first place. It's about recognising that our relationship with food has been an unhealthy one and that we can enjoy our lives without relying on food. We still need pleasure in our lives—we still need that dopamine hit—but it doesn't have to come from food. We can get all the pleasure and emotional support we need from other areas of life. There's nothing wrong with enjoying your food, as long as it's the right food (in our case mega foods), but let's focus on enjoying this great big experience we call life and not just our food. Find something cool to do!

CALORIE DENSITY

Forget about counting, weighing, measuring, controlling, tracking and monitoring your food! Forget about "eat less, move more". Forget about portion control and calorie restriction. Forget about eating in front of a mirror and chewing your food forty-seven times before swallowing. Forget about using smaller plates, eating with chopsticks, placing your fork in the opposite hand or putting your cutlery down in between mouthfuls. Forget about 'mindful eating' and 'mindful fasting'. Forget about waiting until you get hungry and stopping when you're 80% full. Forget about intermittent fasting and "eating windows". Forget about trying to figure out which one of the twelve types of hunger you're feeling right now and how each of these should be handled differently. Forget about not eating after 8pm.

All of these ideas are based on the underlying assumption that there's something wrong with you. There's not. Your appetite is not excessive and you don't need a bunch of unnatural and unnecessary tactics to help you restrain and restrict yourself. You don't need to spend your days being hungry, grumpy and obsessed with numbers, wondering how long you can keep this up.

You can leave these ideas behind now because there's one simple idea that trumps them all: calorie density.

The magic number here is around 600 calories per pound. If you keep the caloric density of your food below this magic number then it's near impossible to eat enough to gain fat. If you want to lose fat, you simply emphasise foods that are lower on the calorie-density scale.

CALORIE DENSITY

Calorie-density refers to the amount of energy in a given volume of food. I like to think of it as calories per mouthful. The Mega Foods Plan is primarily based on foods that are relatively low in calorie density and complemented by other foods that are even lower. This means that you really can eat as much as you feel like, whenever you feel like it, and lose fat without ever going hungry!

Fibre, water and fat content are the three main factors involved here. Fibre and water both contain zero digestible calories, so they take up most of the room in your stomach and make you feel full and satisfied while keeping your caloric intake low. Processed foods and animal products are often very low in water and fibre content, so not only do you get more calories per mouthful but also the exciting nature of these foods means you're driven to consume more mouthfuls.

Fat is a highly concentrated source of calories. Oils are the most calorie-dense foods around while providing next to no nutritional benefit. Yes, that includes olive oil and coconut oil. Meats, dairy and eggs are particularly high in fat while being very low in water content, with no fibre at all. Most people avoid cake and doughnuts, citing "carbs" as their main reason, not realising that the oils, eggs and dairy in their chocolate brownie are contributing the majority of calories in the form of fat.

Nuts, seeds and avocado are natural, health-supporting foods but, owing to their low water and high fat content, they're way above our 600 calories per pound threshold. If you're not trying to lose weight, and you're comfortably able to stop at one handful of nuts per day or a quarter of an avocado (not me!), then go right ahead. If you have trouble limiting your intake of nuts, seeds and avocado, then it might be easier to cut them out entirely. Nutritionally, you won't miss anything in doing this. If you're worried about getting enough "good fats" then add a little ground flax seeds (linseeds) to your mashed potatoes or your bean stew. Problem solved!

Mastering calorie density is mastering food. Everything we do at Spud Fit is aimed at helping you to confidently, calmly and consistently make choices that align with the calorie density model in the long term. Understanding this and getting comfortable with it means that you never have to feel hungry again! This is the backbone of feeling true freedom with food and leaving diet mentality behind forever.

WEIGHT LOSS FOODS	WEIGHT MAINTENANCE FOODS	WEIGHT GAIN FOODS
Unprocessed low-fat plant foods	**Minimally processed and higher fat plant foods**	**Highly processed foods and animal products**
• Potatoes • Sweet Potatoes • Brown Rice • Beans • Bananas • Fresh Fruits • Fresh Veggies etc.	• Wholemeal Pasta • Tofu • Nuts • Avocado • White Rice	• Cheese • Milk • Eggs • Meat (including fish and poultry) • White bread • White pasta • Doughnuts • Chips • Chocolate • Oils - all kinds!

BUT THIS IS HARD

The idea that this is hard or requires extra effort or motivation is the first thing that needs to go. Cooking potatoes is not hard. Take them out of the bag, put them in the oven and come back in an hour. Eating them is not hard either, it's just chewing and swallowing. The only thing that makes any of this hard is the stories we tell ourselves. We need to learn to see through the stories. When we can learn to fully see and accept the reality of our situation, then we can remove emotion from our decision-making process.

This is not a weight loss plan, it's a reality plan. When you fight reality, you will lose every time.

If I get in the boxing ring with Mike Tyson I'm going to get knocked out in about three seconds flat. If someone offers me a billion dollars for surviving one minute in the ring and I work incredibly hard with massive motivation and willpower to get better boxing skills, fitness and strength and really push myself in every way, then maybe, just maybe, I'll last four seconds. Maybe. The point is that no matter what I do or how strong my motivation, if I get in the ring with Mike Tyson I'm going to get knocked out. If I want to avoid getting knocked out, the only logical choice is to stop getting in the ring with Mike Tyson. I have to accept the reality that I'm not a boxer and I just have no chance against one of the all time greats, even if he is well past his prime!

In the same way, a food addict needs to accept the reality that we aren't very good at making spur-of-the-moment decisions with food, and we aren't very good at having "just a little bit, just this once" of any kind of exciting food. The only logical choice is to stop engaging with these behaviours and stop entertaining the illusionary stories we tell ourselves to the contrary. Eating junk food will not relieve your stress or ease your sadness, it will only add to it. This is reality and it does not require willpower to accept it, only logic and rational pragmatism. Pay attention to your thoughts and learn to see the difference between reality and fiction. Based on your past experience, you already know when you're lying to yourself.

MY TWO BIGGEST TIPS:

1.THE 'FIRST EAT POTATOES' RULE

I knew from experience that hunger was always my biggest excuse for giving up on diets. I would justify my choices with something like this: "I was out and about and I was hungry, so I had to hit the nearest fast food restaurant. I had no choice". Of course, this was a load of crap. I could've found some apples at a grocery store if I really wanted to, I was just using hunger as a justification for my poor choices. Nonetheless, I knew that I needed to take this hunger excuse out of play if I wanted any chance at sticking with my Spud Fit Challenge for a whole year.

I decided to never leave the house without potatoes. If I went for a five minute walk to the shop, I took potatoes with me. If I took my son to the playground at the end of our street, I would take potatoes with me. Later on when I started cycling and then running, I would go with a spud in my pocket. In fact it was nearly five months before I left the house for any reason without taking potatoes with me and that was because I was invited to speak at a potato festival where I was pretty sure I'd have no trouble getting food! The point is that if I was out and about and had a hankering for a doughnut, I knew that I'd try to justify to myself by saying: "I had to eat the doughnut because I was hungry." My theory was that if the solution to my hunger was always right there in my backpack, then I'd need to come up with another justification and that might just take long enough to help me see clearly before I made a choice I would regret.

Day four of my Spud Fit Challenge year was rough. I was still in the depths of clinical depression and anxiety and, for whatever reason, that was a particularly bad day. I was driving home in the afternoon, hating the idea of eating another single potato. I was berating myself for having such a stupid, ridiculous idea. "What the hell was I thinking?! Who was I kidding, there was no way that such a hopeless

25

MY TWO BIGGEST TIPS:

loser could achieve such an outlandish thing as eating only potatoes for an entire year!" I'd had enough, and I was ready to throw in the towel and let this become the latest in a long list of failed attempts to gain control over my eating habits.

I was already vegan at the time, so my usual plan was to get two large fries and a large coke. I was embarrassed at my size so I would always get my food and eat in the car where nobody could see me. I'd leave my rubbish in the bin before driving home. I was deeply ashamed of this behaviour and I had to destroy the evidence so my wife wouldn't know what I was doing. As if she would somehow be fooled into thinking I became morbidly obese by sneaking in salads on the way home.

On this day I planned to do the same thing. I pulled into the McDonald's car park and opened the door. As I started getting out of the car, I glanced at the passenger seat and noticed the box of potatoes sitting next to me. Damn. I really wanted to eat McDonald's but I needed to be able to justify it first! All I had to do was eat all the potatoes I had with me so that I could then say "I was hungry and I had no more potatoes with me". My only goal at the time was to bring the hunger excuse back into play. I settled down and started eating. There were at least six, maybe eight, decent-sized spuds in that box. It was a lot of food, and it took some time and effort to get it all down, but I kept going because I wanted that junk food! Fifteen minutes later, I'd finally finished and I was grateful that I could now eat what I was really there for. I opened the door and went to get out again, but this time I was struck by a new and surprising feeling: I didn't actually want McDonald's anymore. There was no debate, I didn't have to talk myself out of it and I didn't have to use any willpower at all! It's easy to say no to something you genuinely don't want! I was confused about what had happened, but I closed the door and continued my drive home anyway.

MY TWO BIGGEST TIPS:

On the way home I realised I didn't want McDonald's for the simple reason that I was already full. This was a massive breakthrough moment for me. I'd stuffed myself with potatoes and, as a result, my cravings had just moved on. The more I thought about it, the more it made sense. There's a reason they feed the sharks at the aquarium before they let you get in the tank with them! By the time I arrived home, the "first eat potatoes" rule was born. I no longer had to tell myself that I could never eat junk food again. I no longer needed to do battle with my inner demons telling me why I needed to eat an entire packet of cookies on the way home from grocery shopping. Instead, I could say "no problem, you can eat whatever you like—just fill up on potatoes first and then see how you feel" and invariably the craving would be gone. Since then, this has worked for me time and time again.

It's important to note that this is not about having a small snack. It's about getting seriously full before making decisions about junk food. When I finished my Spud Fit Challenge year, I kept following this same rule but using Mega Foods as well as potatoes. The 'first eat potatoes or other healthy, whole, unprocessed plant foods' rule didn't quite have the same ring to it, so I decided to stick with the 'first eat potatoes' rule.'

Most importantly, if you don't have potatoes with you all the time, then this rule will not work! Don't forget that you can replace potatoes with other healthy, whole, unprocessed plant foods. Bananas are a great example of a handy food on the go. Buy a big bunch, eat the lot, then get on with your day.

MY TWO BIGGEST TIPS:

2. THE CRAVINGS GYM

As long as Mandy and I have been together, the top shelf of the fridge door has always been where we keep our chocolate. I had no intention of asking Mandy to change the way she did things for me. As far as I was concerned, this was my problem and it was up to me to find my own solution. If I was living alone then I wouldn't have chocolate or other junk foods in the house. I would keep my own environment pristine; after all, it would be silly to buy food that I had no intention of ever eating. This was not my situation and I did not want to impose myself on my family in any kind of limiting way.

For the first few days of my Spud Fit Challenge year, I viewed that chocolate shelf as my nemesis. The thought of reaching past the chocolates to get a potato from the fridge made me nervous and I thought it was only a matter of time until I couldn't stand it anymore.

Sometime during week two, I went for a walk to the shop to buy more spuds and I got to thinking about this uncomfortable chocolate shelf situation. I needed to find a way to get better at dealing with my cravings because I knew that it was only a matter of time before my willpower gave way, and I found myself inhaling a family-sized block of irresistible chocolate and chasing it down with a litre of coke.

My history as a former elite athlete means that I tend to use sport as a term of reference for a lot of things in life. I wanted so badly to get better at dealing with the cravings that were constantly triggered by the chocolate shelf. On that walk I thought about how, if I ever wanted to get better at any aspect of my sport, the answer was always very simple: practise. If I wanted to get better at running then I had to go running. If I wanted to get stronger, then I had to lift heavy things.

MY TWO BIGGEST TIPS:

If I wanted to improve a skill, then I had to do drills. Suddenly the answer was obvious - if I wanted to get better at dealing with cravings, then I had to practise! I had to intentionally put myself in situations where cravings would arise and challenge me.

Even the best, most successful athletes in the world have days when they really don't feel like going to the gym. It's hard work, it's going to hurt, it's going to be sweaty and uncomfortable. It's certainly not going to be as nice as hitting the alarm and going back to sleep! Despite these things, I've never heard of a single person who managed to drag themselves out of bed and get to the gym to smash out a solid training session and then regret putting in that effort. Every single person who has ever gone to the gym has had days when they'd rather stay in bed, while nobody has ever regretted making the effort.

From that moment forward, I decided to stop looking at the chocolate shelf as a thorn in my side and, instead, to see it as an opportunity to practise. The chocolate shelf was no longer my nemesis, it was my cravings gym! Before going to the fridge for potatoes, I would take thirty seconds and talk myself through it: "This is going to be uncomfortable, it might even hurt a little and I'm probably not going to enjoy it. I'd rather avoid it completely. But I know that when I'm finished, I'll be glad I stuck to my guns and I'll be proud of getting through a tough situation. Best of all, my cravings-resistance muscle will be a little bit stronger than it was before".

The 'cravings gym' mentality is something I have since aimed to cultivate in all areas of my life. Whatever challenges you face, learn to see them as opportunities for growth instead. Doing hard things makes us physically and mentally stronger. The reverse is also true. Be grateful that people and the environment around you are providing you with chances to practise and strengthen your cravings-resistance muscle. After all, if you can't practise then how will you improve?

DON'T THINK, DO!

We waste so much time and energy on planning, preparing and researching. We wonder about the best ways to buy, prepare, store and eat food. We play out a million different scenarios in our minds, imagining how we'll resist food temptations at work, book club meetings, that wedding next month, the holiday cruise etc.

The more we think, plan and answer questions, the more we come to understand that there are some questions that can't be answered. We can't possibly account for every situation that could arise and we are kidding ourselves if we try.

On top of our logistical and tactical worries come the intrinsic questions regarding willpower, motivation and self-worth. Probably the most common thing I hear is some variation of "I hope I can do it". We all have plans and dreams, an idea of what our perfect life would be like.

We have lists of things we're desperate to achieve, if only we could figure out X, Y and Z first.

I'm here to tell you that none of the above matters. Not in the slightest. Most of our questions and worries only serve to do one thing - slow us down.

Can I do this for a week, a month, a year?
Can I eat well at my sister's birthday party next month?
What about that vacation?
What will people say?
Will I get too bored?
Do I have the willpower?
Do I have the motivation?
Am I strong enough?

DON'T THINK, DO!

The honest answer to these questions and many more is very simple - "I don't know." There is no truthful way to answer any of these questions until you reach the moment where you get to find out for yourself.

Don't borrow problems from the future, you have enough on your plate (pun intended!) to deal with right now.

Stop asking yourself unanswerable questions and stick with one that you absolutely can answer - Is it possible for my next meal to be a healthy one?

The answer to this is so simple and easy that the question almost seems silly. Of course it's possible for you to eat a healthy breakfast, so go and do it! Right now it really doesn't matter if your breakfast in seventy-eight days from now will be healthy or not, so forget about that and ask yourself instead - can my next meal be a good one? Of course it can, make it so!

Stop thinking and start doing. You will most definitely make mistakes along the way; no amount of thought or preparation will stop that from happening. The average Olympic figure skater falls around 10,000 times in training before we get to watch them on TV. You are going to fall too and you're also going to get back up and learn from it.

Action is all that matters. Don't think, DO!

EXERCISE

Eat less, move more has been drummed into us all for decades. We've covered how to eat less (calories) while actually eating more food, which in my opinion is the best thing about the Mega Foods Plan! Now it's time to take a brief moment to talk about exercise.

When most people think about getting healthier and losing weight, the first thing that comes to mind is joining the gym or going for a run. Move more seems like the easiest and most obvious part of the equation to tackle first. So we join the gym where we hate the music, feel intimidated by all the ridiculously fit people and can't understand how all the machines work and what the hell a superset is. Then there's the alarm clock screaming at us at 5am and the three extra coffees we need to help us get through the day. Worst of all is after a couple of weeks we feel sore, tired and drained, without even losing any weight!

If you're exercising to lose weight, you're barking up the wrong tree! Let me explain. The average woman needs around 2000 calories a day just to live her life. To create a calorie deficit (eat less), she might adopt a strict calorie counting diet that allows her 1500 calories per day, giving a 500 calorie deficit. She might then include exercise that burns 500 calories per day, thereby increasing her calorie deficit to 1000 calories! The problem is that the increased deficit also means she will have increased hunger, which leads to increased stress, tiredness and grumpiness and makes it close to impossible for her to stick with this plan for an extended period.

Now, let's put the same woman on the Mega Foods Plan. She follows the rules of this plan, eats as much as she wants to at all times and pays attention to the principles of calorie density to naturally end up eating around 1500 calories per

EXERCISE

day. When she adds in the 500 calories worth of exercise, her hunger drive increases in the same way, but instead of allowing herself to get extra hungry, tired and grumpy, she just eats more because she feels like it. She will probably go very close to eating an extra 500 calories per day to compensate for the exercise! This approach makes it more sustainable because she doesn't have to battle with the hunger demon all day long.

So, if exercise doesn't make a huge difference in weight loss, what's the point?! Moving your body, increasing your heart rate, working your muscles and getting a sweat on is healthy for so many reasons. Improved heart and lung (cardiovascular) health are two obvious ones, with exercise shown to help lower blood pressure and resting heart rate among other things. Exercise helps maintain and even increase bone mass and density, which is very important as we age. It helps lower blood cholesterol and can help with managing diabetes.

This list could go on and on but, in my opinion, the most important thing about exercise is the way it can help improve our mental health. First, a decent bout of exercise releases endorphins and 'feel good' hormones that can improve your mood and flow on to improve your productivity, relationships and feelings of self-worth. Second, one of the best ways to build pride and self-esteem is to do hard things. Exercise is hard, and there's a feeling of pride and confidence that comes with knowing that you've pushed yourself and managed to get your exercise in, even though the couch was singing you sweet lullabies!

The million dollar question now is what's the best kind of exercise? The best exercise is the one you can repeat often. Just like with food, we need to make the healthy choice the easy choice. So, choose an exercise that you like doing and start with that.

EXERCISE

Bonus points if you can do it with friends who will make it more fun but also keep you accountable. Think of an activity that you used to like but might've let slip. Don't be afraid to experiment and try new things. Don't worry if you no longer like the things you used to do. If you're not sure where to start, get an audio book and go for a walk. There's a phone app called Audible, which will give you a free trial. I only allow myself to watch action movies (which my wife Mandy can't stand) when I'm on our indoor rower. This trick works every time!

I want to stress that, in the beginning, you should forget about exercise entirely. It's hard enough to overhaul your diet without the added pressure of needing to get your 10,000 steps in! As you continue along the Mega Foods path, you'll notice that your energy levels start increasing and you'll arrive at a point where you just feel itchy to move. That's the time to start.

FAQ

Q: *Can I eat as much as I like?*

A: You can and you should! Eating less than you would like to means that you will need to rely on willpower to stick with it. It also means going hungry and dealing with the stress, anxiety and grumpiness that comes with it, not to mention the fact that your brain is literally powered by carbs. For most of us it's not sustainable to be hungry all the time, so we are better off eating in a way that allows us to eat as much as we feel like, as often as we feel like it.

Q: *Can I **really** eat as much as I like?*

A: Yes! Re-read the calorie density section to understand why and how this works.

Q: *Can I combine this with one meal a day, intermittent fasting?*

A: For most of us, eating one meal a day and other types of intermittent fasting creates unnecessary hunger, stress and rules that are made to be broken! Fasting can help you lose weight quicker, but it also relies on willpower to get you through and creates extra opportunities to fail and give up. Long-term sustainable changes in behaviour are more achievable when we remove as many obstacles as possible. Suffering through hunger is certainly a huge obstacle for most of us!

Q: *Is it ok to eat after 8pm?*

A: Maybe you'll play with this as a self-experiment at a later date, but the time of day is irrelevant at this point in your journey. There is no bad time to eat good food!

FAQ

Q: *How much water should I drink?*

A: There is no correct amount of water to drink daily. The aim of drinking water is to stay well hydrated, and you can't tell if you're well hydrated just by measuring how much you drink. The easiest way to tell if you're well hydrated is to check the colour of your urine. If it's clear or very pale yellow then you're all good, and if it's yellow then you're dehydrated. I suggest following a very simple process: 1) Drink as much water as you feel like throughout the day. 2) If you notice that your urine is yellow, have a big glass of water or two straight away. Easy! Your water consumption will naturally increase through this way of eating anyway.

Q: *What supplements should I take?*

A: On the Mega Foods Plan there should be no need for any supplements other than B12. This important vitamin is produced by bacteria that's often found in dirt. Modern improvements in hygiene have improved human health in a myriad of ways, but it's also meant that we now unintentionally eat far less dirt than we used to because we wash our food (and our hands) far more thoroughly than we used to. It's theoretically possible to get enough B12 if you grow your own organic veggies and don't wash them too thoroughly. I'd rather be on the safe side with this one though.

If you are unable to spend at least 15 minutes in direct sunlight each day then you should also consider a vitamin D supplement, especially in winter.

FAQ

Q: *What kitchen gear do I need? Do you have a favourite?*

A: All you need is a way to make food hot. That could be a stove, oven, microwave, campfire, etc. My most used item is our pressure cooker. It's great because it's so easy to just throw in some spuds, add a cup of water, press the rice button and come back a bit later to lovely, steamed spuds. We have a couple of good quality non-stick pans in different sizes and a high quality set of knives. Our air fryer also gets a workout most days.

Q: *What if I fall off the wagon?*

A: Language matters. The first thing to do is recognise that you didn't fall and there is no wagon. You also didn't slip or trip or come unstuck. Nobody pushed you, nobody forced a doughnut into your mouth against your will, you simply made a choice. When you can accept full responsibility for your choices then you can also accept that you are capable of making different choices. You are in charge; you have full control over this situation. Best of all there is no wagon and it is not getting away from you while you ponder the next step, so you don't have to worry about catching up to it. Just make the next choice a good one—start with eating a spud!

Q: *Is salt ok?*

A: Salt in itself is not bad but the way we use it is a big problem in the standard western diet. Fast foods and packaged foods generally contain excessive salt. Restaurants and cafes tend to use a lot of salt too because it's delicious and exciting and will keep you coming back for more.

If we cook with salt, we can use quite a lot and the flavour still tends to get lost in the process. Then we need to add more salt after we serve the food. If you never

FAQ

use salt in cooking and instead just sprinkle a bit on your food once it's on the plate, the salt will be the first thing to hit your tongue and you'll get the full flavour. Using salt in this way is self-limiting - if you use too much then it gets overpowering pretty quickly and you won't want to eat it.

If you have heart disease or another specific problem that you're dealing with then you might want to avoid salt completely; otherwise, if you follow this method you'll stay below the daily recommended limit.

Note that commercial stock powders and many other herb and spice mixes often contain a significant amount of salt.

Q: *Are smoothies ok?*
A: Depending on who you ask in the whole food plant based world, smoothies could be a nutritional gold mine that will supercharge your mind, body and spirit OR they could be just another way of getting too many calories, too quickly.

I think both ideas are true, so I take a couple of simple steps. I got into drinking smoothies because my kids like them. It's a really simple, easy and delicious way to get some greens into them without resistance and we have fun making them together. So most days we make smoothies and we talk about all the great fruits and veggies that go into them and how they help us.

I think it's best if we chew our food rather than have a machine do that for us, but I've also got no chance of getting my kids to sit down to a big plate of everything that goes into a smoothie. To stop myself from getting too many calories, too quickly, I do two things:I drink with a straw and I have it while I'm doing something else. I might sip it while I'm at my computer or cleaning the kitchen for example.

FAQ

This way I take it in very slowly, and I end up drinking far less than if I just gulped it down straight from the blender jug.

Q: *Is cane sugar ok?*
A: People also ask about raw sugar, brown sugar, coconut sugar and maple syrup. These are all essentially the same thing - highly concentrated calories with little nutritional value. If you'd like to use a teeny tiny amount to give a little flavour to your oats then go for it, but please don't fall into the trap of thinking that one is healthier than the other.

I try to use whole fruits as natural sweeteners when it makes sense. For example, I make porridge with a mashed banana and some chopped dates: could life get any sweeter than that?!

Q: *Is bread ok?*
A: Bread is better than ok, it's great! Bread made from minimally processed, ground whole grains with all of their wonderful fibre will support your health in many different ways. Use it to make a salad sandwich full of veggies and hummus (see our Spud Fit hummus recipe later in this book) and you've got a perfect meal that ticks all the boxes.

By now it goes without saying that you should check the ingredients to make sure your bread has no added oils or sugars and uses only whole grains. This sort of bread is easier to find in some parts of the world than others, so if you're desperate for the convenience of bread, you might have to consider making it. Otherwise, rely instead on potatoes, grains and other mega foods.

Additionally, some people find it hard to stop eating bread once they start. If that's you then you might be better off leaving it out, at least until you reach your goal weight. Same goes for wholemeal pasta.

Q: *Is rice ok?*

A: A couple of billion or so fit, healthy, lean Asian people have thrived into old age on a rice-heavy diet for millennia. A big bowl of rice and veggies is an excellent way to get a plethora of nutrients in a single meal while giving you the fuel to dominate your day. White rice is fine, if that's all you can get, but I recommend going for the extra fibre in brown rice whenever possible.

Q: *Is fruit ok?*

A: Many people complain that fruit makes you fat because of the sugar content. If you read the calorie density section earlier, you'll understand that the high water and fibre content in fruit means that they're actually a low-calorie density food that will support your weight loss goals and your health. The only caveat for me is that fruit doesn't tend to keep us feeling as full for as long as starchy foods like spuds, rice and beans.

I don't put a limit on how much fruit you can eat but, from my experience, most people do better when they focus on emphasising starchy foods. It's up to you to experiment and figure out what feels good to you. Pay attention to how it makes you feel, how your hunger fluctuates throughout the day and adjust accordingly.

Q: *Do I have to buy organic??*

A: Let's not complicate things too much. Your number one goal should be to eat unprocessed, whole plant foods and exclude everything else as much as humanly possible. You should do everything you can to make that as simple as you can. If eating organic is too expensive for you, or you have to travel too far to get it, then conventionally grown food will do the job perfectly well. Eating organic food is nice for a variety of reasons, but the last thing we want is for you to throw your hands in the air with frustration over the extra expense, effort and time that might be required for you to make this work.

FOREWORD TO THE RECIPES

Recipe books are usually a chance for a chef to show you how to create a cacophony of gastronomic splendour that will delight and impress your family and friends and leave you wishing you didn't go back for that third helping. That's NOT this book! This is real life, where we just need to get a good healthy meal on the table quickly and easily, several times a day, every day, forever. These recipes won't be the most delicious meals you've ever eaten, but that's not the point. We're here to help you free up your time, brain space, energy and money while putting yummy, ridiculously healthy food on the table for you and your family.

Continually chasing the next 'high' that comes with rich and exciting food concoctions is likely a big part of the reason you're reading this book right now. It's time to move on from that mindset! Our food is flavourful, hearty and satisfying, but it won't give you that big dopamine spike that you're used to getting from food. It's tasty because we're not about total deprivation, we all know that doesn't work. It's okay to enjoy your food but it's not ok to have it dominate your life, and it's not your fault you've been suffering with that. Our first goal here is to help you feel satisfied while achieving your peak physical condition without stressing about what, when, where, why and how to eat.

Above all else we need to stay focused on making the healthy choice the easy choice. This means doing the basics on a consistent basis. It's a very rare occasion that you can look in our fridge and not find a box of cooked potato and a box of cooked rice. There's often some cooked beans in there too. This makes it super quick and easy to throw a meal together and have it on the table inside ten minutes if you want to. It's also uncommon for me to leave the house without taking food. I might grab a couple of cooked spuds, a bag of apples or a bunch of bananas on my way out the door. Maybe some leftover mashed potatoes or another meal if I'm

FOREWORD TO THE RECIPES

going somewhere with a microwave. Sometimes we go out for a short time and it turns into a long time. I don't like being hungry and the temptation that comes with it, so I do what I can to avoid that situation. If I do happen to get caught short on my food supply when I'm out, I keep in mind that most of the time I'm not far from a supermarket or fruit and veg shop. A kilo of grapes makes a great meal in a pinch.

Try to relax and experiment. Don't let fear stop you from giving things a try and experimenting with flavours and ideas. The worst thing that can happen is some food goes in the bin but that's highly unlikely. Or that one meal is a bit less delicious than you'd like it to be, but so what? You don't have to follow our recipes perfectly. We don't! Play with them, change cooking times and experiment with flavours until you find the best way for you.

Simplicity is a major factor in the continued success of just about everyone who loses weight and keeps it off. This won't work because you got better at cooking or you stumbled upon the most amazing recipes, it will work because you accepted that there's more to life. It will work because you understand that as long as your belly is full of good food, everything else you need to live your best life is already inside you. I hope this book helps you free up some time and energy to bring your best self to the surface.

RECIPES - NOTES FROM MANDY

When I created the recipes for our first book, The DIY Spud Fit Challenge, I didn't include measurements for any of the ingredients. The point of both of our programs is to get to know yourself, to really start to understand your relationship with food. Where do *you* have to draw the line, where do *you* need set limitations and boundaries to keep it interesting enough to be able to stick to the plan, but not so tasty and interesting that it sends you spiralling back into the old habits that no longer serve *you*? However, I understand that it's helpful to have guidance, and so in this book I have simply written out the recipes as I made them in a particular moment in time. They're rough measurements. I change them around every time, because I just guess as I go. Goodness knows I'm no chef, I'm just making healthy meals that my family and I will enjoy. If you don't like capsicum, leave it out. If you want to put in a whole jar of onion powder instead of a teaspoon, well frankly I don't blame you, ha!

Same goes for serving sizes. On both the Spud Fit Challenge and Mega Foods Plan, you are probably going to eat a lot more food than you've ever been 'allowed' on any diet you've tried. To that end, most of the recipes are created for one meal, for one person. The others you can decide for yourself whether or not you want to share or save the leftovers for your next meal.

Many of the recipes call for 'cooked potatoes', or 'cooked rice'. You should always have your preferred staples cooked and ready to go in the fridge. If not, you'll need to cook them before you start the recipe, according to the instructions on the packet.

The Porridge Cookies, Mash Chips and 'Nice-cream' all work better when left to set overnight. The others can be prepared as you need them.

RECIPES - NOTES FROM MANDY

Equipment. As Andrew has already said, you don't need any special equipment, just a way to make your food hot. That said, we have found a pressure cooker particularly handy for this way of abundant, healthy eating. An air fryer is another investment we're glad we made, and that we use every single day.

Herbs and spices: go to town! This is the perfect opportunity to try tastes and flavours you may never have tried before, or to try old flavours in new ways. Remember to take it easy on stock powder to keep sodium content low.

Finally, when you've moved to the Mega Foods Plan, don't forget the magic of the mono-meal. It's perfectly healthy - and very freeing - to eat a meal that consists only of watermelon or bananas...or potatoes!

We really hope you enjoy these recipes and make them your own! We'd also love to hear about the quick, easy and healthy Mega Foods meals you include on your menu. Please feel free to share them with us by emailing the recipe and pic to andrew@spudfit.com or mandy@spudfit.com, and let us know if we have permission to share publicly.

Eat simply. Live fully!

Andrew and Mandy

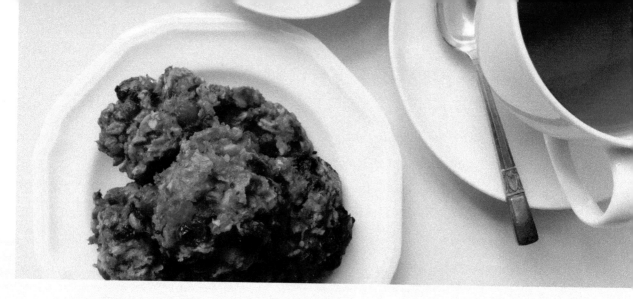

We're always looking for ways to simplify our food and make the right choice the easy choice. This recipe is a perfect example of that: delicious, comforting porridge now, but even better later when you need a sweet, filling and convenient snack on the go!

PORRIDGE (AKA OATMEAL) COOKIES

Ingredients

3 ripe bananas

5 cups oats

1 cup sultanas

1 tablespoon ground flax (linseed)

3 cups water

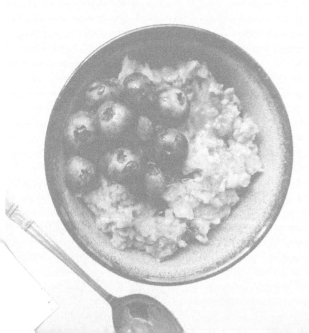

Directions

Mash the bananas in a big mixing bowl.

Add the other ingredients and mix until you get the consistency of thick porridge. Adjust water as necessary.

Cook in the microwave or on the stovetop according to packet instructions.

Eat a bowl for your breakfast!

Transfer the leftovers to a container and refrigerate for several hours or overnight.

When the porridge is set, use a spoon to scoop the mixture into cookie-size chunks and place them directly into your airfryer.

Heat on high/200°C/392°F for approximately 11 minutes, or bake on a tray in your oven at 200°C/392°F for approximately 40 minutes.

All the classic fry-up veggies in one huge, satisfying bowl! You need pre-cooked spuds for this recipe, so grab them from the stash you already have ready to go in your fridge.

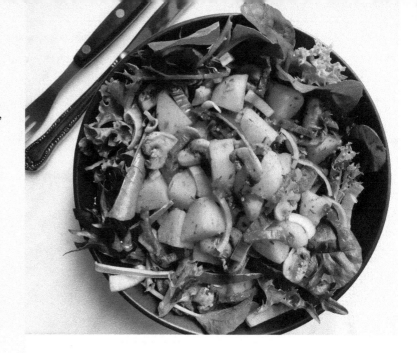

BIG BREKKY SALAD!

Ingredients

2 boiled or baked potatoes, diced
1 cup white or brown mushrooms, chopped
2-4 handfuls mixed salad greens
¼ red onion, finely chopped
¼ cup oil-free sun-dried tomatoes, finely chopped
1 teaspoon onion powder
1-2 teaspoons spice blend of your choice

For the dressing

Choice of either:
1 tablespoon lemon juice, mixed with 1 teaspoon Dijon mustard (optional), OR Balsamic vinegar

Note: We use a commercial 'roast potato' blend of onion powder, garlic powder, paprika, thyme, oregano, ginger, ground coriander, pepper, caraway seed, mustard seed, and nutmeg. Moroccan spices are also delicious, and of course you can always prepare your own!

Directions

In a non-stick pan add 1/4 cup of water then add mushrooms and fry for one minute. Do not add oil.

Add onion powder and spice mix, stir, then diced potatoes with a little more water so it doesn't dry out. Stir again to cover potatoes with onion powder and spice mix, cover and steam for 1-2 minutes.

Arrange all the salad greens in a big bowl.

When mushrooms are cooked and spuds heated through, add them to the greens.

Add chopped red onion and sun-dried tomatoes.

Mix thoroughly and add dressing.

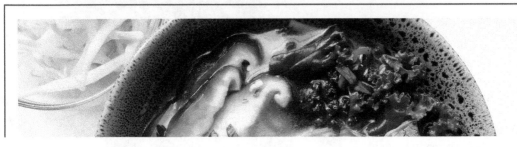

PHÔ-INSPIRED BREAKFAST SOUP

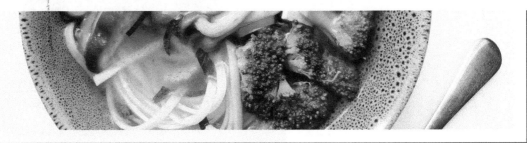

Some of us just prefer savoury breakfasts! I am one of those people. I've been hooked on Phô, a traditional Vietnamese breakfast dish, since I first tried it. It usually takes a very long time to make. This is my quick, easy and super simple Mega Foods version.

Directions

In a medium saucepan, bring 700ml (23½ fl oz) water to the boil.

Add noodles and cook for the time stated on the packet. Add other ingredients in the following order accordingly:

Add mushrooms in final three minutes.

Add broccoli in final two minutes.

Add leafy greens and tofu/tempeh in final minute. If using fresh ginger, add this too.

In a very large bowl, pour desired amount of water from the saucepan to form the broth, and drain off the rest.

To the broth add onion powder, powdered ginger, vegetable stock, minced chilli peppers (if used) and mix.

Add the rest of the contents of the saucepan to the bowl.

Squeeze over lemon juice and top with fresh coriander, mint, bean shoots, sriracha/hot sauce and fresh chilli.

Ingredients

100g (3½ oz) brown rice/buckwheat/other whole grain noodles
½ - 1 cup mushrooms, chopped (your choice, I love a pre-packed blend of oyster, shiitake etc.)
½ head broccoli, cut into half-florets
2 large handfuls leafy greens such as kale, bok choy, silverbeet (chard), chopped
½-1 teaspoon onion powder
¼-½ teaspoon ginger (fresh, minced or powdered)
¼-½ teaspoon salt-reduced vegetable stock
Juice of ¼ lemon

Optional:
- 50 g (2 oz) shaved firm tofu or tempeh (I shave with a potato peeler to create very thin pieces, you can also chop into blocks)
- minced chilli peppers to taste

To garnish:
- fresh coriander and/or Vietnamese mint
- sriracha or other oil-free hot sauce
- handful fresh bean shoots
- fresh chilli peppers, chopped

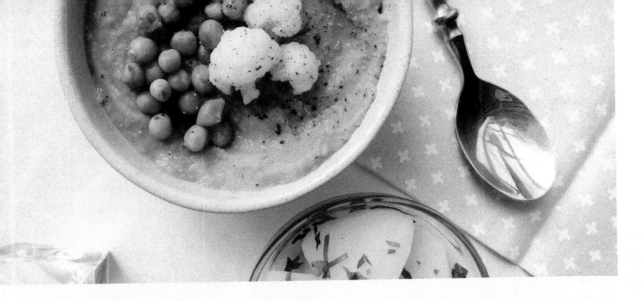

I was raised on pea soup and my whole family absolutely loves this recipe. Warming, filling, tasty and packed with an abundance of vitamins and minerals - not to mention it costs about $2 to feed the whole family. It's got it all!

SUPER SIMPLE SMOKY SPLIT PEA SOUP

Ingredients

1 packet dried green split peas

½ cup fresh or frozen chopped brown onion

1 cup frozen green peas

1 tablespoon onion powder

1 teaspoon salt-reduced vegetable stock powder

1 teaspoon smoked paprika

Optional:

Other riced/very finely chopped veggies as desired. We use a frozen riced broccoli/cauliflower/sweet potato mix to increase the veggie content.

Directions

If you have a pressure cooker, such as an Instant Pot, simply place all ingredients into the pot, add water as per instructions on dried peas packet, stir, select 'soup' setting and press start.

If you are cooking on the stove:

In a large pot, water fry chopped onion for 1 minute.

Add dried peas and water according to instructions on packet. Add stock, onion powder and smoked paprika. Add extra veggies, if using.

Stir well, then occasionally while cooking according to the dried peas packet (usually simmer for around 20 minutes).

Eat as is, pour over boiled potatoes or have potatoes as a side in place of bread.

Cooked fruit. Some people hate it. We can't get enough of it! As with all of our recipes, feel free to eat as much of this as you want. If you're trying to gain or maintain weight rather than losing, you can add a few cashews too.

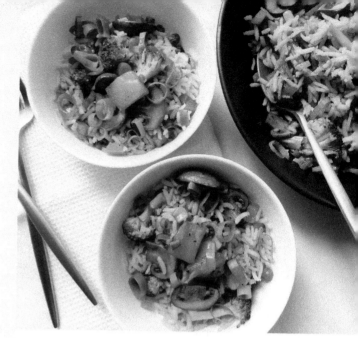

ABUNDANT PINEAPPLE FRIED RICE

Ingredients

3 cups uncooked/6 cups pre-cooked brown rice (we always have a stash pre-cooked)
1 cup fresh or frozen cauliflower/broccoli florets
½ cup red capsicum (bell pepper), chopped
½ cup pineapple pieces in juice (retain juice)
½ cup mushrooms of your choice, chopped
½ cup frozen peas and corn mix
½ cup fresh or frozen brown onion, chopped

1 teaspoon fresh/minced/powdered garlic
1 teaspoon onion powder
1 teaspoon fresh/minced/powered ginger

To garnish:
1 spring onion (scallion/green onion), chopped
Fresh coriander
Salt-reduced soy sauce (minimal, to taste)
Fresh chilli
Lime juice

Directions

If using uncooked rice, cook this first in a rice cooker or pressure cooker, or on the stove in a large pot of water according to packet instructions (usually equal parts rice and water, boiled for 12 minutes).

In a large non-stick wok or fry pan, add the pineapple juice plus enough water to make about 1 cup of liquid in total.

Add brown onion, powdered onion, garlic and ginger. Stir fry on high for 30 seconds.

Add mushrooms, broccoli and cauliflower, capsicum (bell pepper), peas and corn, and finally pineapple pieces. Stir fry for another 3-5 minutes. You may need to add very small amounts of water at a time - you don't want it to dry out but you don't want it too soggy either.

Add cooked rice, mix thoroughly and heat through.

Serve topped with minimal soy sauce to taste, chopped spring onions and fresh chilli.

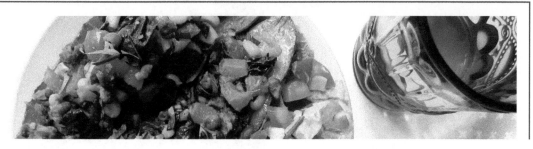

MEXICAN-STYLE LOADED SWEET POTATO

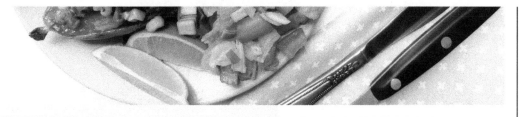

This dish really needs no introduction. Simple, satisfying and just enough excitement!

Directions

Pierce sweet potatoes all over with a fork. Bake at 220°C/425°F for 40-45 mins, until tender.

Meanwhile, in a large non-stick pan heat half a cup of water, the onion and vegetable stock powder. Add black beans, peas, corn and capsicum and cook for 3 minutes.

When the sweet potatoes are ready, slice down the middle and top with cooked beans and veggies, fresh veggies and top with fresh coriander. Squeeze over fresh lime to taste.

Ingredients

1 large baked sweet potato (or more!)
1 cup canned black beans (or more!)
½ cup each of:
- fresh or frozen peas and corn
- red capsicum (bell pepper), chopped
- fresh tomato, chopped
- iceberg lettuce, chopped
- baby spinach or other leafy green of choice, chopped
¼ red onion, finely chopped
¼ teaspoon vegetable stock powder
¼ teaspoon onion powder
¼ cup fresh coriander (cilantro), chopped
Juice of fresh lime

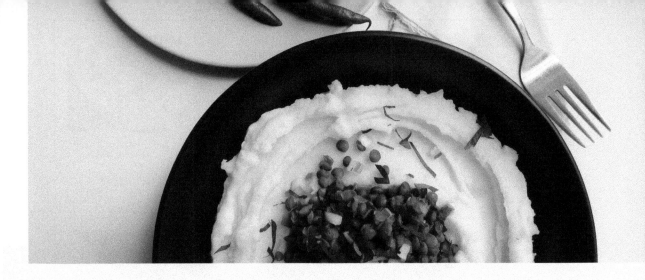

Leave it to the French to inspire something so perfectly simple
and perfectly elegant at the same time!

FRENCH LENTILS WITH MASH AND GREEN BEANS

Ingredients

400g (14oz) canned French/Puy/brown lentils (you
can also cook from dried if you want to reduce salt
as the cans usually have salt added)

½ brown onion, chopped

1 stick celery, diced

1 small carrot, diced

2 cloves garlic, crushed (or use minced or
powdered)

½ teaspoon onion powder

½ teaspoon vegetable stock powder

½ teaspoon Dijon mustard

1 teaspoon dried or fresh 'French herbs' - we like a
blend of parsley, tarragon, sage, rosemary and
thyme.

On the side:

Large handful fresh green beans, topped and tailed,
or broccoli florets or other greens of your choice,
steamed.

Juice of fresh lemon

Directions

Make mashed potatoes as per recipe on page
55, cover and set aside.

In a non-stick pan fry ½ a cup of water, the
brown onion, celery, carrot, stock powder,
onion powder and mustard for 2 minutes,
stirring well. Add more water as necessary to
avoid drying out and sticking.

Drain lentils and add to the pan with herbs.
Stir to mix, and cook for a further 3 minutes
or until carrots and celery are soft.

Meanwhile, blanche or steam your greens to
desired texture.

On a plate add the mash and top with the
lentils. Serve the greens on the side with a
squeeze of lemon juice.

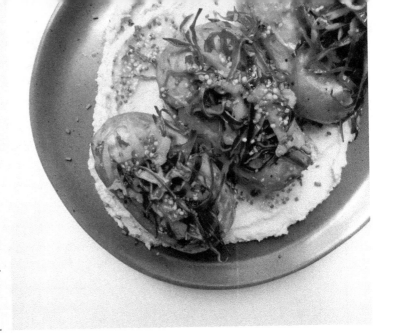

This book would not be complete without this absolute classic. Enjoy and enjoy again!

LOADED SPUD

Ingredients

2-3 large spuds
2 cups coleslaw veggies, either pre-packed (discard dressings/toppings) or homemade (see below for recipe).
¼-½ red onion, chopped
¼ cup chives, chopped

For the dressing, mix:
1 tablespoon fresh lemon juice
¼ teaspoon Dijon mustard
Add water for volume

To top:
¼-½ cup hummus (as per our recipe, page 57, or source a commercial oil-free, tahini free low-fat version)
Balsamic vinegar (or other fat-free dressing/sauce of your choice)

Homemade coleslaw:
½ cup purple cabbage, finely shredded
½ cup white cabbage (savoy is great), finely shredded
½ cup carrot, finely shredded
½ cup apple, finely shredded

Directions

Preheat the oven and bake potatoes at 180°C/356°F for 90 mins (or as long as it takes for the knife to come out clean if you poke them). You can also microwave them, however, they won't be as tasty or crunchy on the outside/fluffy on the inside.

If you are making your own coleslaw, now is the time to prepare it. Hand mix the finely shredded cabbage, carrot, and apple (or use the pre-packed coleslaw). Mix and pour over the lemon juice, mustard, and water dressing and mix thoroughly through the coleslaw.

Remove potatoes from the oven and slice open.

Top with a big dollop of hummus (¼-½ cup), lots of fresh slaw and the chives.

Finish with balsamic vinegar or other fat-free dressing/sauce of your choice.

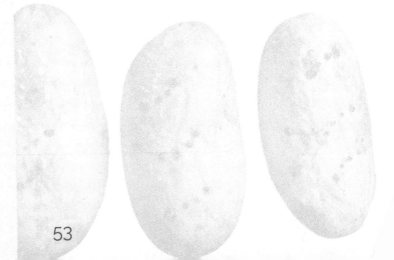

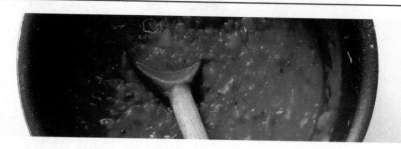

LENTIL MUSHROOM BOLOGNESE

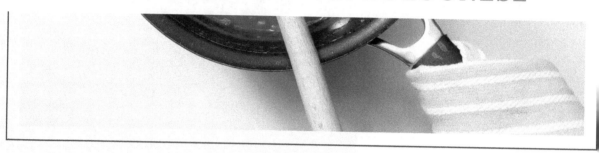

Andrew's specialty! This is something the whole family will love.

Directions

In a large non-stick pot, fry garlic, onion, carrot, celery and mushrooms in quarter of a cup of water on high heat until onion is translucent (2-3 mins). Add a splash of water here and there to prevent drying out.

Add remaining ingredients and simmer on medium heat for 10 mins.

Serve over a baked white or sweet potato.

Ingredients

400g (14oz) canned brown lentils
2 cups mushrooms, diced
1 carrot, diced
1 stick celery, diced
1 brown onion, chopped
3 cloves crushed fresh or 1 heaped teaspoon minced garlic to taste
½ cup oil-free sundried/semi-sundried tomatoes, chopped
3 cups (24fl oz) jar of passato (tomato puree)
2 teaspoons dried Italian herb blend (or fresh herbs to taste, try basil, oregano, parsley, thyme)
1 teaspoon vegetable stock powder

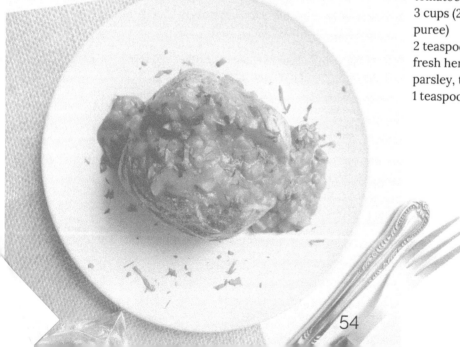

This seems complicated because of the overnight step. However the key is to make a huge batch so that you have delicious, steamy, fresh mashed potatoes for dinner and then keep the leftovers to make these mash chips tomorrow! That way you get two different meals out of one pretty simple preparation.

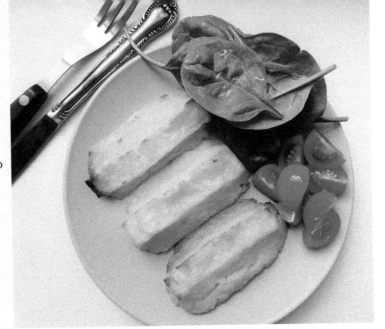

MASH/
MASH CHIPS

Ingredients

3 - 4 kgs (6.5 - 9 lbs) potatoes (less if you don't have a big enough pot)
1 tablespoon onion powder
2 teaspoons garlic powder
1 tablespoon vegetable stock powder
2 heaped tablespoons nutritional yeast
1-2 cups (8-16 fl oz) low-fat (oil-free) soy, oat, rice or other plant milk of your preference.

Notes: You need just enough milk to achieve your desired consistency for mashed potatoes. Usually 1-2 cups is enough for me, depending on which spuds I use. You can also use water if you don't want to use milk.

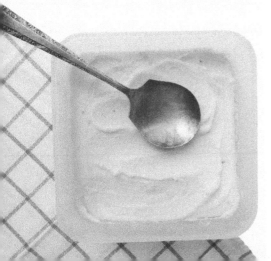

Directions

Put your potatoes in a large pot and cover with water. Bring to the boil and cook for 30-40 minutes, or until you can easily stick a knife in and pull it straight out again. Alternatively, you can use a pressure cooker: add the potatoes and a cup of water, hit the 'rice' setting and press go.

When they're ready, drain the water. Add all ingredients except the milk to the pot and mash thoroughly, slowly adding milk every so often until you achieve your desired consistency.

Serve and enjoy a delicious meal of mashed potatoes, maybe with some other veggies too.

Now it's time for Mash Chips!

Put the leftovers in a box, spreading them out so the top is as level and smooth as possible. Store in the fridge overnight to set.

When they're set firmly, tip the box upside down on a chopping board and tap on the box so that your mash falls out as one big block.

Using a long, sharp knife, cut your mash block into thick 'chips'.

Place the chips into the air fryer, making sure to keep them separated. Cook for 10 - 15 minutes, depending on your desired crunchiness. Best to check a few times to be sure they aren't burnt.

If you don't have an airfryer, you can bake on an oven tray lined with baking paper for 15-20 minutes, turning them 2-3 times.

Yet another option is to slice into 'hash brown' shapes and fry in a non-stick pan to make 'mash browns'!

This is a game changer. No it doesn't taste exactly like dairy cheese, but it's tasty and satisfying - and unlike dairy cheese - the more you eat the healthier you'll get! Use it on everything.

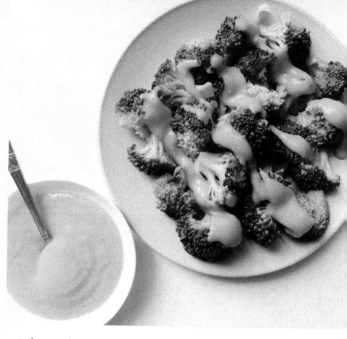

POTATO & CARROT 'CHEESE' SAUCE

Ingredients

3 potatoes, quartered
2 carrots, quartered
1-2 tablespoons nutritional yeast
1 heaped teaspoon onion powder
1 heaped teaspoon vegetable stock powder
1 level teaspoon smoked paprika
1/2 - 1 cup (4-8oz) oil-free plant based milk

Directions

Boil potatoes and carrots together until both are soft (approximately 20 mins).

Drain and add to a blender with ½ a cup (4oz) of milk and remaining dry ingredients.

Blend until smooth, adding remaining milk as necessary to achieve preferred consistency.

Serve over baked potatoes, steamed veggies or use as a dip for a raw vegetable platter!

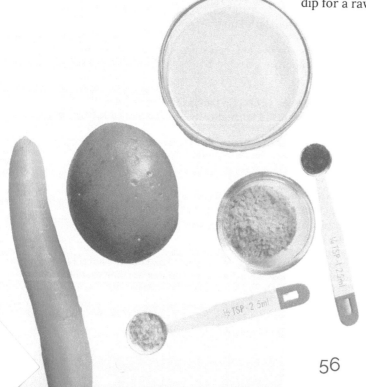

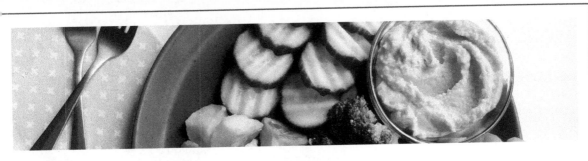

HUMMUS

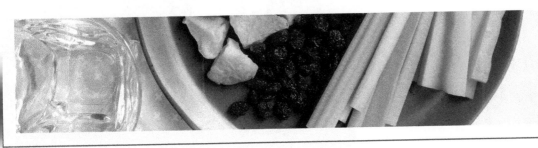

However much hummus you usually eat, it's not enough!

Directions

Drain the liquid (aquafaba) from two cans of chickpeas into a bowl and set this aside. Leave the aquafaba in the third can with the chickpeas and add this and the other two cans of drained chickpeas to a high speed blender.

Add remaining ingredients to the blender and blend everything until smooth and creamy, stopping to mix and scrape from sides as necessary. Add small amounts of the saved aquafaba if you need it to stop the mixture becoming too thick. Discard leftover aquafaba once you've achieved your desired consistency.

Serve the hummus in a bowl with your favourite dipping veggies. I go for sticks of carrot, capsicum (bell peppers) and celery. You can also flavour your hummus with a wide variety of spices, or add fresh herbs, and/or top with hot sauce for a bit of a kick!

I also like this hummus served on a baked spud with some broccoli.

Under no circumstances should you share this with your work colleagues!

Ingredients

3 cans (approximately 1.3kg/3lbs) chickpeas
1 heaped teaspoon onion powder
1 heaped teaspoon vegetable stock powder
1 teaspoon smoked paprika
Juice of 1 lemon

Sweet tooths, this is your moment! Really fill up on this satisfying sweet bowl of goodness, and your secret junk food stash will lose its appeal.

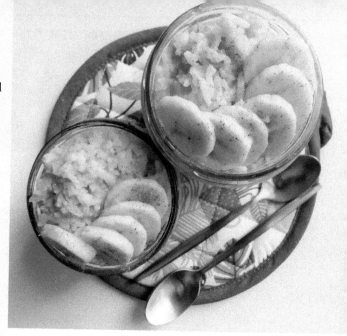

SUPER COMFORTING RICE PUDDING

Ingredients

2-3 cups cooked rice of choice (we like a mix of brown, black, red and white)
1 - 1½ cups (8-12oz) oil-free plant-based milk of choice
½-1 cup fresh fruit (banana, berries etc.)
¼ teaspoon vanilla essence or extract
Nutmeg/cinnamon or your choice of sweet spice blend to taste
A few drops of maple syrup to sweeten if desired

Notes: We always have a batch of staples such as rice ready to go in a container in our fridge. If you don't have cooked rice ready to go, you can cook from scratch according to packet instructions, or buy pre-cooked rice - but make sure it's oil-free!

Directions

Combine rice, milk, vanilla, spices and fruit in a medium saucepan and cook on medium heat for 3-5 minutes or until heated through. You can also heat in the microwave.

If you prefer, leave the fruit raw as a topping instead of cooking it.

Sweeten with a few drops of maple syrup, if that fits within your plans for yourself.

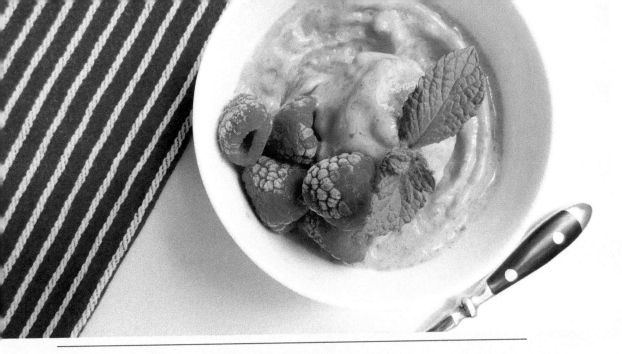

'NICE'-CREAM

Nice for your tastebuds, even nicer for the rest of you.
Move over ice-cream, we have nice-cream now.

Ingredients

4 bananas, peeled and frozen

1 cup frozen berries, mango or other fruit of choice

(you can buy frozen or buy fresh and freeze

yourself)

¼ teaspoon vanilla essence

Nutmeg/cinnamon or other sweet spice mix to

taste

Splash of oil-free plant-based milk of choice

Directions

Add all ingredients to a blender, only adding milk as necessary to achieve your desired 'nice'-cream consistency (do this very slowly to avoid adding too much!).

You can eat straight away but this recipe works even better if you leave it to freeze overnight.

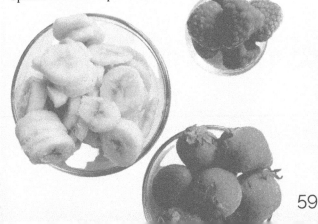

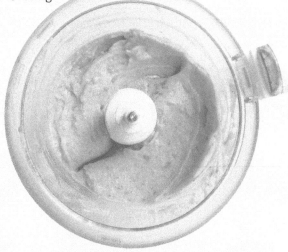

LIST OF CONTRIBUTORS

Many people were enormously generous in providing us with help and support to get this project off the ground. Without them I have no doubt that this book would still be an idea bouncing around the in the back of my mind, and perpetually stuck near the bottom of my to do list. There are many more people who chose not to be listed here, I can't thank you all enough for your kindness, thoughtfulness and patience.

Joe Jacob	Mary Harris	Laura Woodson
Marty Ritz	Elly Emmett	Paul Manzanero
Jan Koprek	Nic Potter - Plant Based Nic	Laura Tlougan
Kent Hugosson	Julie Simiana	Daniel Fernández
Lily Blue	Kym Mulvey	Georgia DeLeon
Nicole Bathurst	Mary-Jeanne Smith	Tamsin Young
Jen Dickman	Sherri MacLean	Jennifer Noonan
Bruce Guernsey	Jamila Hassan	Ashleigh Gauch
Dayna Ferreira	Kim Castrillon	Coral Horton
Katie Downing	Angela Peerman	Suzannah Troy
Loz Miller	Joanne Kiele	Jennifer Bilodeau
Christine (Chris) Prevost	Donna Womer	Jae-Samantha Forest
Wendy Skiba-King	Diane French	Sheila Yount
Christopher Monk	Lynne Powell	Laurie Ellington
Connie Adderly		

ACKNOWLEDGEMENTS

Special thanks go to Paula Banda for her amazing food styling and photography. My daily meals taste great but look like they were dropped from a significant height with great aim to land in my bowl. I enjoy eating them but I'm sure my readers wouldn't enjoy looking at them! Paula has made our food look every bit as great as it makes me feel. Please check out her work at www.anewgreenleaf.com or on Instagram @anewgreenleafofficial.

My jumble of words, overuse of commas and general malaise and indifference towards the correct anaphoric use of pronouns was thoroughly snapped into line by the grammatical maven know as Amanda Holder. Thanks for guidance in turning this P.E. teachers' incoherent musings into a literary masterpiece, half of my future Pulitzer prize will belong to you. Get in touch with Amanda via her email: amandaholdereditingservices@gmail.com

Thanks most of all to my dream woman, Mandy van Zanen, for being the greatest cheerleader the world has ever known. Without you, my greatest achievement in life would be figuring out that I can save 10 seconds every morning by using elastic laces so I don't have to tie my shoes when I leave the house. With you in my corner, the impossible becomes probable and that's before you even start with the pompoms and high kicks.

Thank you all.
Andrew

CPSIA information can be obtained
at www.ICGtesting.com
Printed in the USA
BVHW011032190522
637508BV00009B/282